BROUGHT TO EARTH BY BIRTH

Harriette Hartigan

Motherbaby Press

Motherbaby Press
An Imprint of Midwifery Today
PO Box 2672
Eugene, OR 97402-0223
USA
(541) 344-7438
Fax (541) 344-1422
mbpress@midwiferytoday.com
motherbabypress.com
midwiferytoday.com

Cover and interior design: Cathy Guy
Front cover image: Harriette Hartigan

ISBN: ISBN 978-1-890-44642-0

Printed and bound in the United States of America

For more information:
motherbabypress.com/books/BirthPhotos.asp

A NOTE TO YOU...

Spirals weaving throughout these pages
are from pregnancy itself.
They are improvisations I discovered while
exploring the photograph on page 16.

Cathy Guy, wonderful graphic designer
at Motherbaby Press, improvised my spirals
into a lovely motif, which you see flowing
among the photographs and words.

The spirals feel like whispers to me,
of beauty and grace within
pregnancy's magnificent nature.

"THERE IS NO OTHER PLACE
OF WHICH ONE CAN SAY WITH CERTAINTY
THAT ONE HAS ALREADY BEEN THERE."

Sigmund Freud

CONTENTS

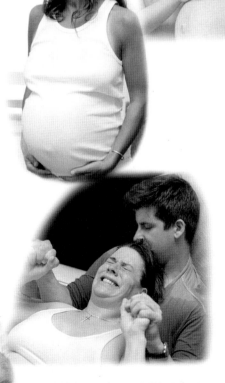

DEDICATED

to my sons, John, Zay and George, and their father, John.
You encouraged me with abiding belief in the value of what
I was creating, from the very beginning when pregnancy
and birth were seldom seen. I treasure your trust
and love, deeply in my heart, beyond words.

ACKNOWLEDGEMENTS

Like grains of sand along the shore,

numerous are those who have taught and guided me

on the path that brings this book into your hands.

Each birthing woman and her family

whom I've photographed, midwifed and interviewed;

Midwives, nurses, doctors and childbirth educators with whom I've worked;

Friends and colleagues who grace me by their presence in my life

and with their expertise—here are a few who reflect the many not named.

Carol Bower suggested that I photograph her pregnancy in 1973.

Barbara Henning invited me to photograph her birth in 1975.

Esther Broner said, "You will write about this!" and mentored me.

Linda Honey's profound trust in birth taught me also to trust.

Kitty Ernst midwifes me into the future.

Jamie Bolane's early publication of my work was valuable.

Rahima Baldwin Dancy's thoughtful challenges keep me evolving.

Jane Arnold's insightful epiphanies move me on.

Sloane Crawford has been my midwife colleague through many births.

Timothy Johnson's enthusiastic appreciation is abiding.

Teri Shilling's support and teaching ideas delight me.

Elizabeth Shadigian's wise inquiries and care mean so much.

Mickey Sperlich skillfully edited when it was time.

Jan Tritten created Motherbaby Press, devoted to wholesome birthing, supported by her exceptional staff.

My life and work is blessed by each of you. Thank you!

INVITATION

This book is potent.
I suggest you take it to
a quiet place without disturbance
of phone, television or computer.

Absorb its power and grace.
Birth, of eternal significance,
is celebrated with insight, art
and reverence for the power of creation,
which joins us together in life here on earth.

Open your heart and mind to
the images and words.
Go within yourself,
to birth itself—
this intimate realm of being.

Jan Tritten

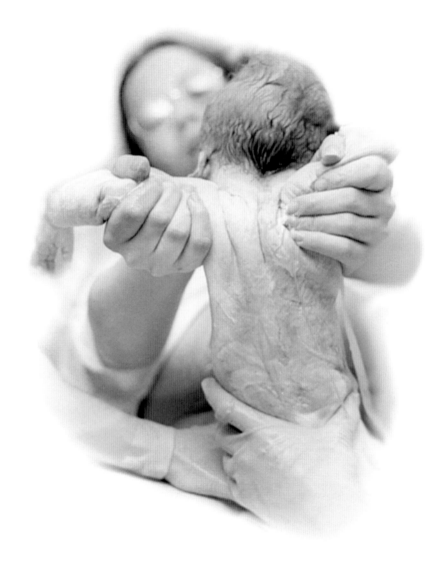

CREATION

BIRTH IS THE EXPERIENCE OF A LIFETIME

Giving birth and being born bring us into the essence of creation,

where the human spirit is courageous and bold

and the body, a miracle of wisdom.

Nobility, epic and ancient, radiates through women

as they live the sensual beauty of their pregnant bodies

and open with magnificent strength to birth's profound imperative.

And we the newborns journey persistently, insistently through women's bodies,

to this earth, in the power of primal energy.

The experience of birth is vast. It is a diverse tapestry woven by

cultural customs, shaped in personal choices, affected by

biological factors, marked by political circumstances.

Yet the nature of birth itself prevails in

elegant design of simple complexity.

Perhaps this is also our deepest metaphor

as we continue to birth throughout life,

opening to the new and unknown,

living the effort of becoming.

FACING THE MYSTERIES OF CREATION AGAIN AND AGAIN

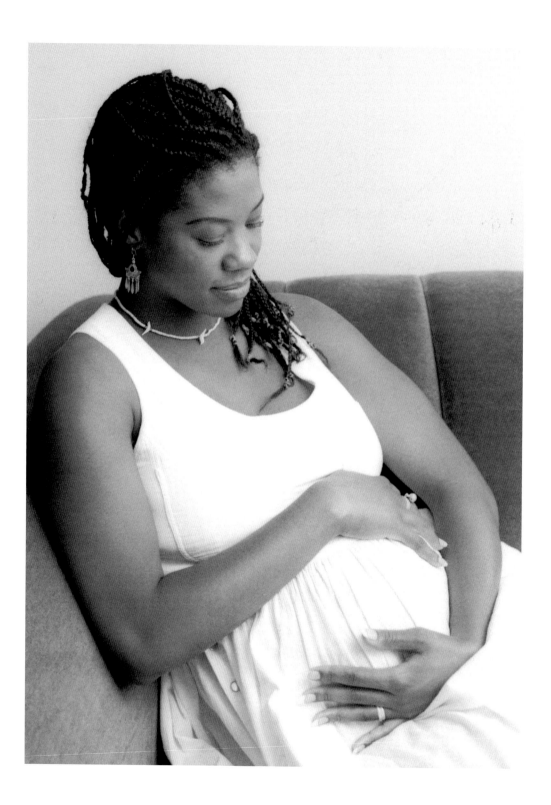

THROUGH THE LENS

BIRTH IS WORTHY OF OUR SIGHT

Women ask me to photograph their pregnancy and
birth experiences, knowing that what they accomplish is without equivalent.
There is longing to see again and again, and to remember.
Photographs bring to sight what has been lived
and give time to ponder details.

Diane recalled what she was thinking during the intensity
of labor, as she looked at her birth photographs.
"There's a power, a force. I am a woman. I can do it."

Ruth said, "I fell in love with my husband all over again," when she
looked for the first time at the photographs of Dan holding her in labor.

"That's me, that's me!" said three-year-old Linee pointing
to her newborn self in the family album.

"I think it's in all of us to know birth,"
whispered a dad, looking back with tears
at the moment his daughter was born.

IT IS A DEEP PRIVILEGE TO PHOTOGRAPH BIRTH

I am guided by the reverence and awe one feels in the presence of the sacred.
Here are portraits of dignity and grace within the midst of splendid, passionate work.
Moments of significance are framed by powerful efforts of labor
and the exquisite truth of birth.

Brought to Earth by Birth is a poem of my reflections
through years of photographing birth,
attending as a midwife, and continually witnessing
this elemental reality we all share.

These photographs are intimate but not private.
Women and families are sharing their personal moments.
I am very grateful for their generosity and trust.
Feel free to accept their gifts.

I INVITE YOU THROUGH THE LENS TO BIRTH'S SPACES/PLACES
WHERE IMAGINATION ENTERS AND MEMORY ROAMS

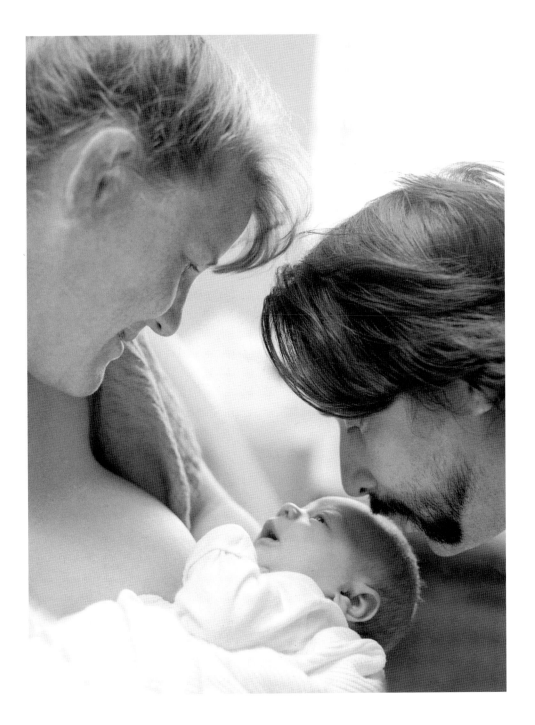

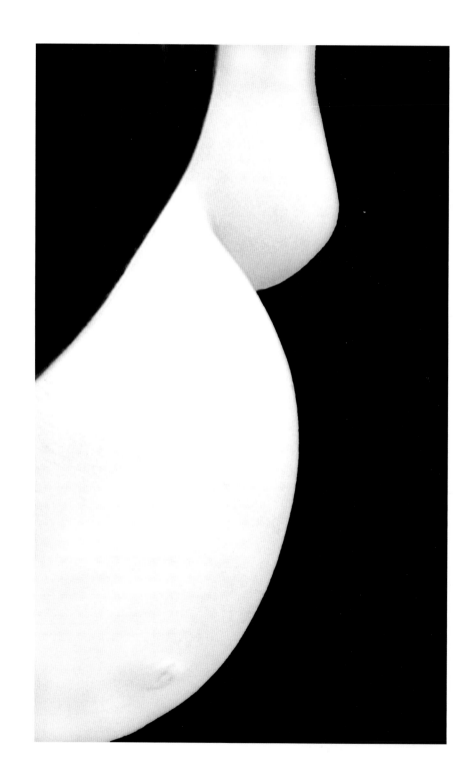

PREGNANCY

In pregnancy's sculptured beauty,
one body grows within another.
Energy becomes human in the
alchemy of the womb.

Cells multiply, change and grow.
Within woman's body, the
heartbeat of another life pulses.

Emotions delight and perplex.
Wonder. Worry. Certainty. Doubt. Love. Fear. Joy. Anger.
Passion. Excitement. Feeling vulnerable. Feeling powerful.

Ambivalence is response
to the gift and the responsibility.

Pregnant woman,
at once universal and individual,
lives the compelling force of creation
within her whole being.

FIRST HOME...BODY ITSELF

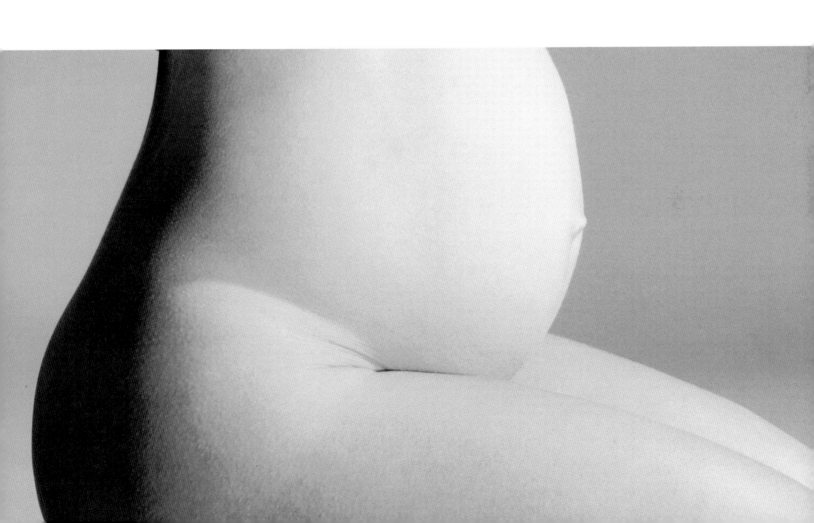

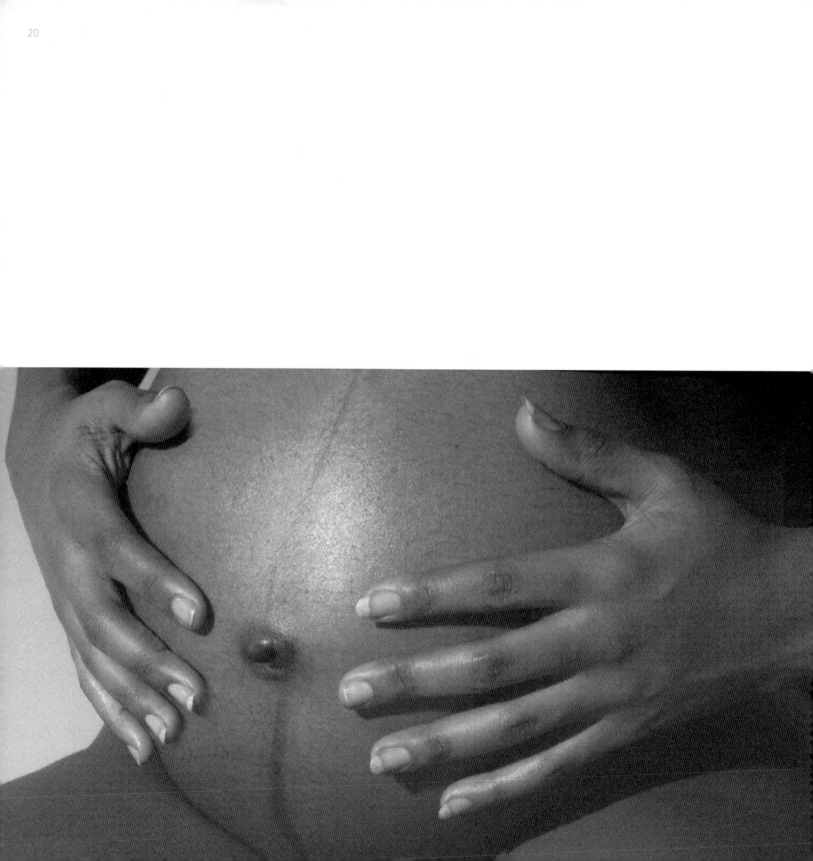

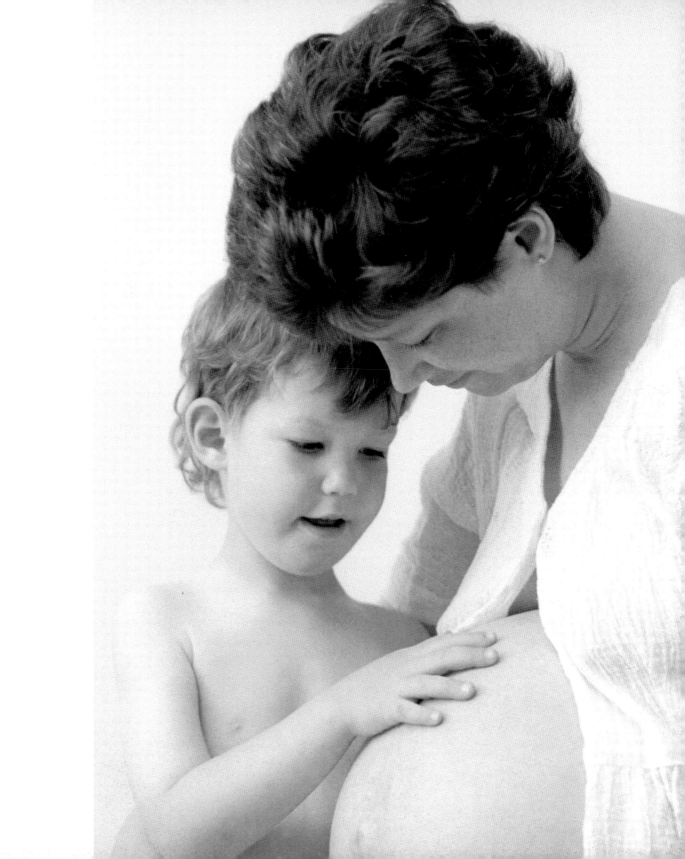

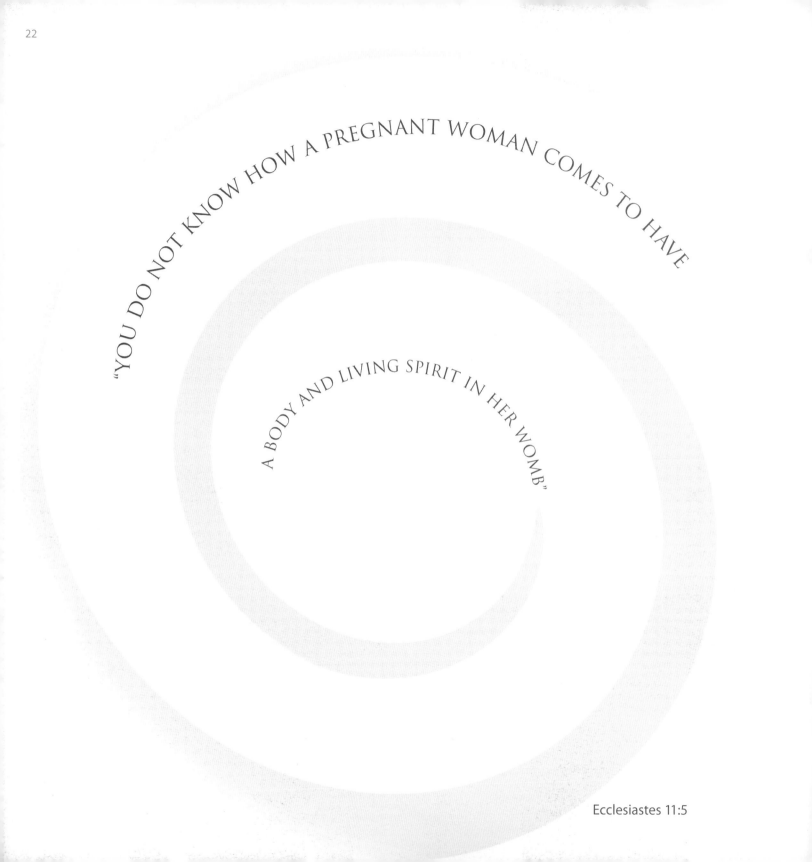

"YOU DO NOT KNOW HOW A PREGNANT WOMAN COMES TO HAVE

A BODY AND LIVING SPIRIT IN HER WOMB"

Ecclesiastes 11:5

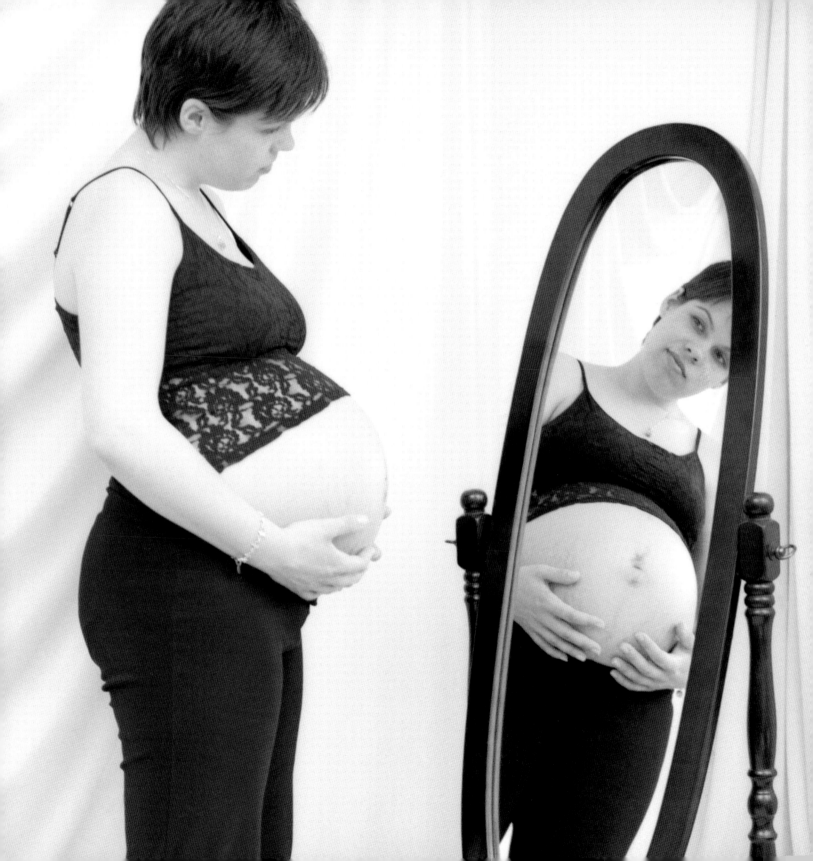

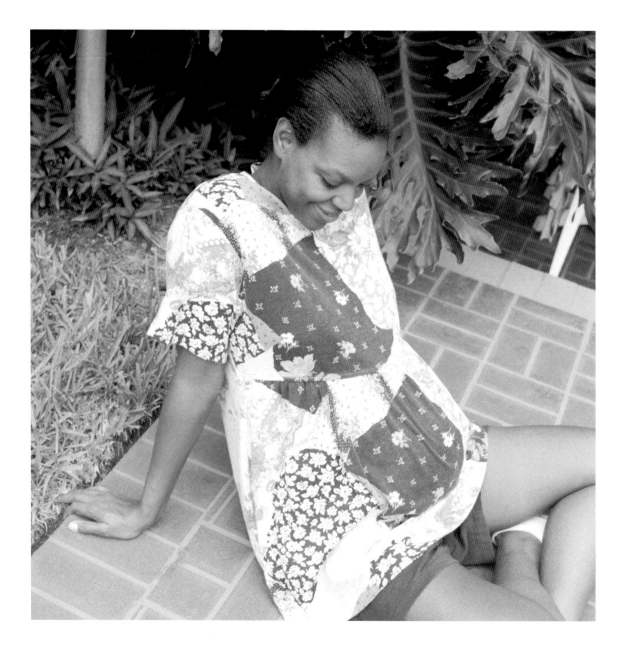

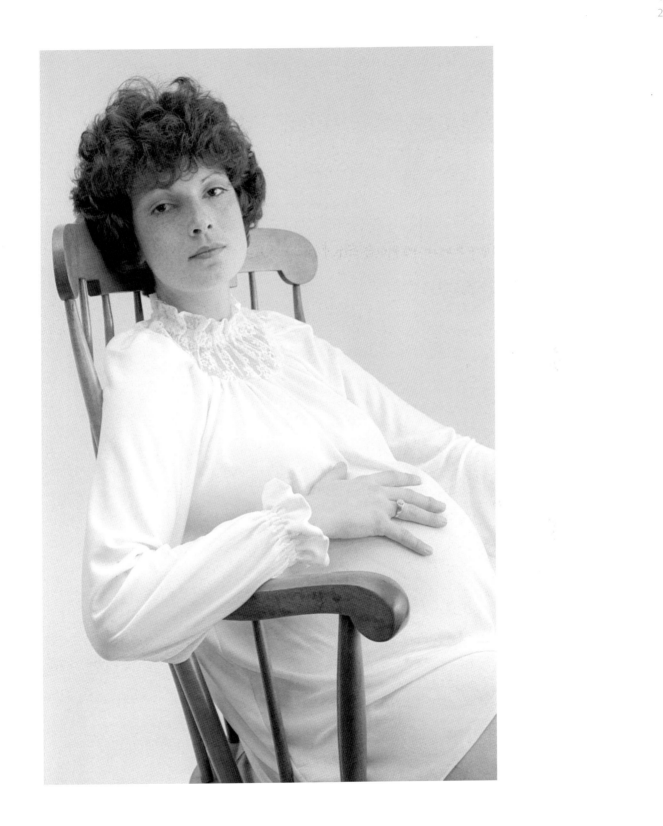

" ...SONGS OF THE BODY

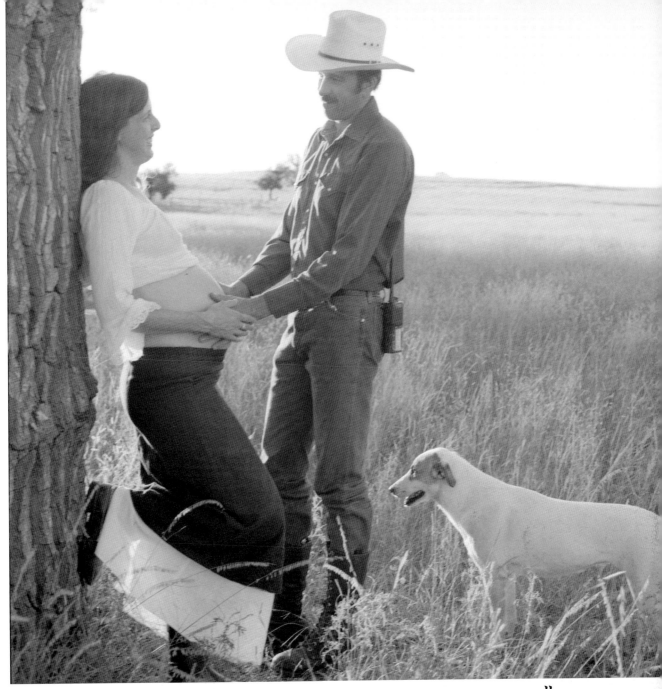

AND OF THE TRUTHS OF EARTH." Walt Whitman

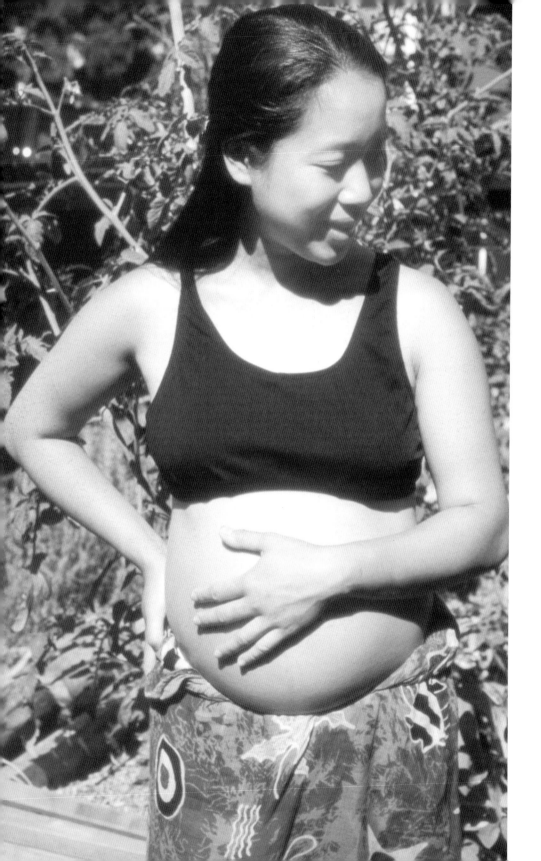

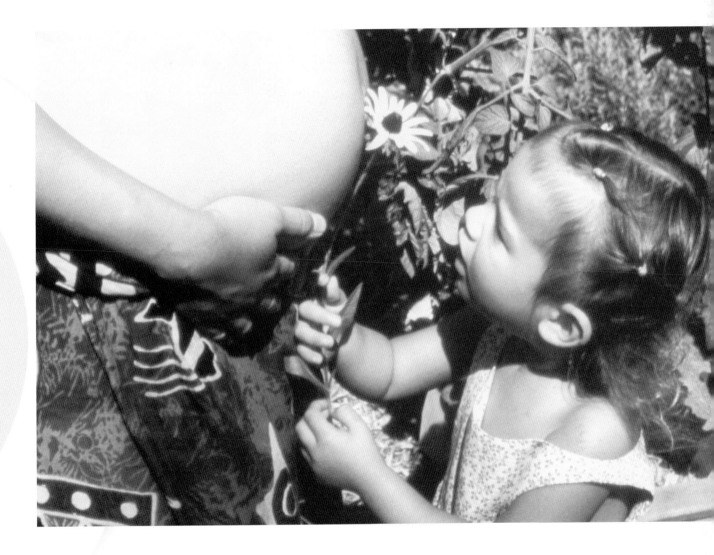

living

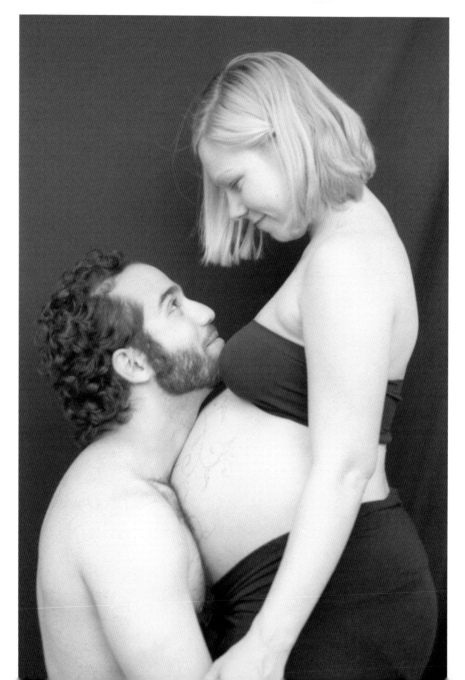

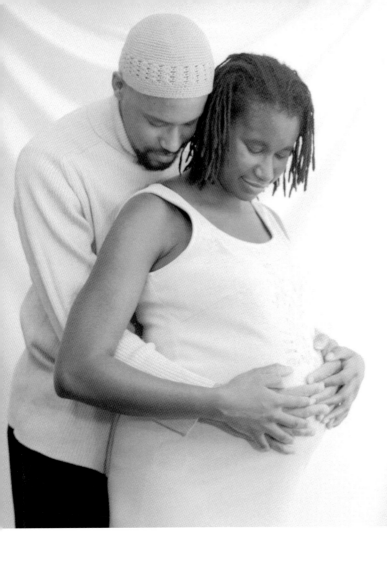

the experience

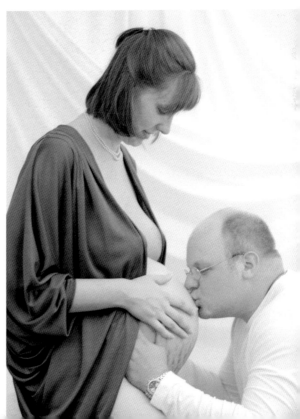

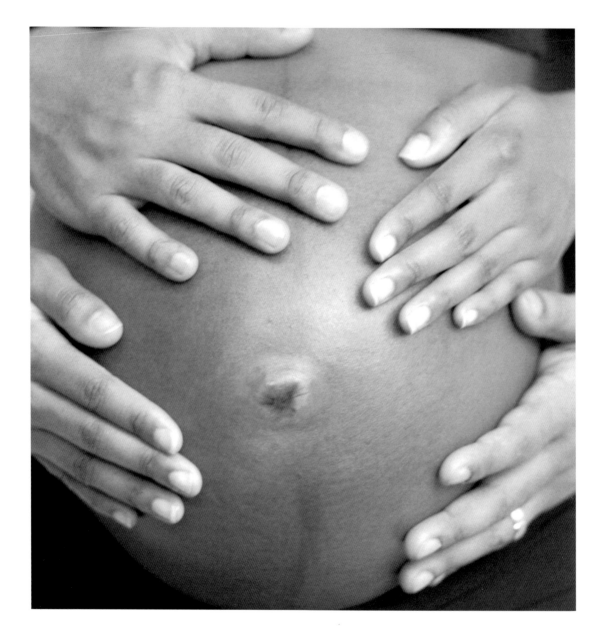

THE WONDER OF MONA LISA'S SMILE

the essence of her mysterious expression,

is ancient reflection of woman

pondering new life within.

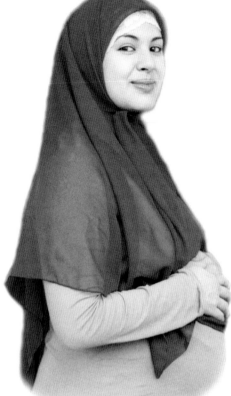

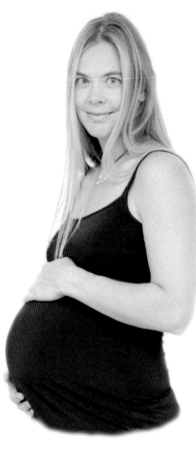

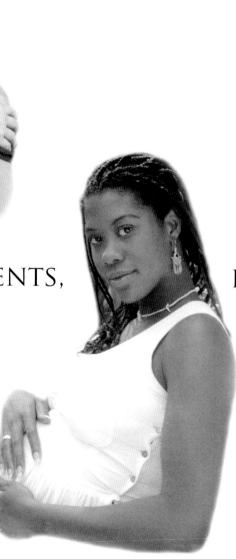

MONA LISA MOMENTS, LIVING THE MYSTERY

OPENING TO THE POWER

Borderland

a realm between
earth & birth

where only birthing woman goes.

WITH THE GRACE OF MYSTERIOUS TIMING

pregnancy ends and labor begins.

We do not understand what starts the dynamic process of labor,

yet the wisdom of two bodies, mother and babe, know.

The uterus, strongest muscle in the human body, contracts with absorbing persistence.

In giving herself to the power, birthing woman opens fully, instincts ancient and accurate.

Intensity from this enormous effort stretches consciousness beyond language,

to a borderland marked by relentless emotional and physical sensations.

Doubt that she can do this mighty work,

and determination that "Yes, I will," are both true.

Family and friends give comforting words of encouragement,

and touch her with love. Care providers offer their skill and expertise.

These sustain birthing woman in the

solitary work that only she can do.

LABOR

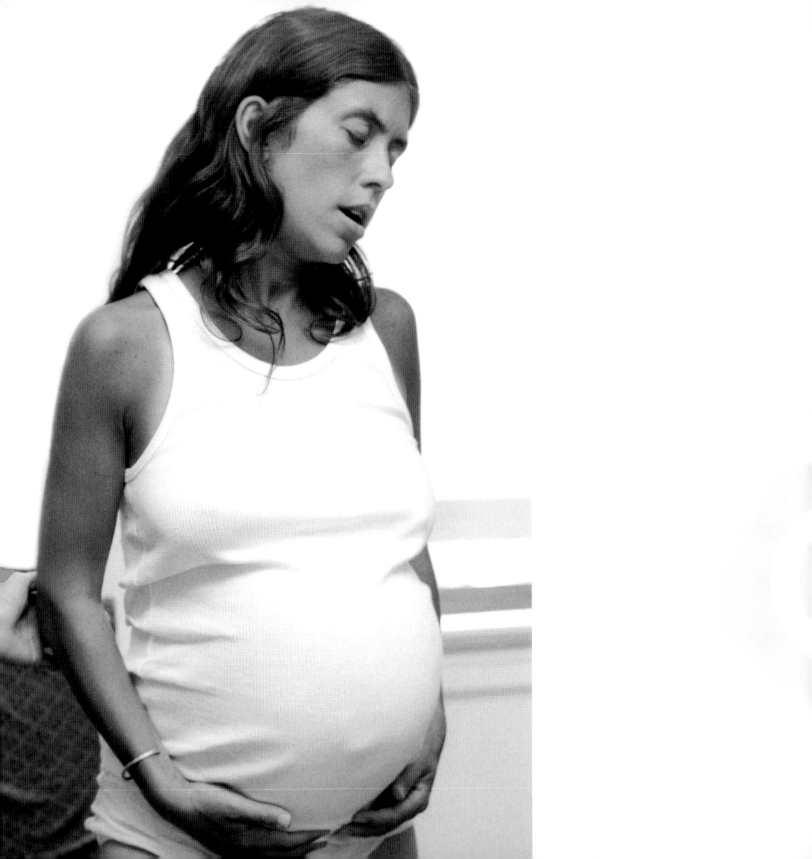

"EVERY CELL IN MY BODY WAS BUSY, COMPLETELY,

UTTERLY OCCUPIED WITH THE EFFORT OF BIRTHING."

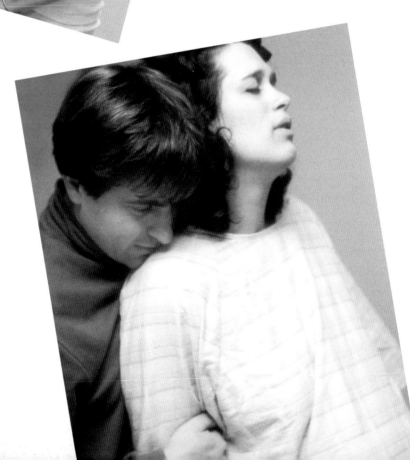

"THEY SAID I SEEMED SO CALM,

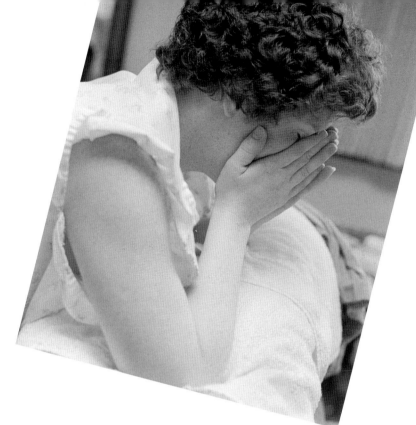

BUT MY MIND WAS WHIRLING…
BODY TAKING OFF."

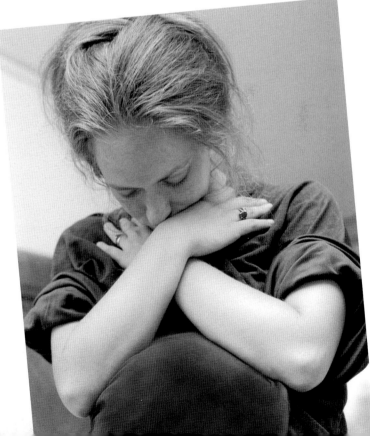

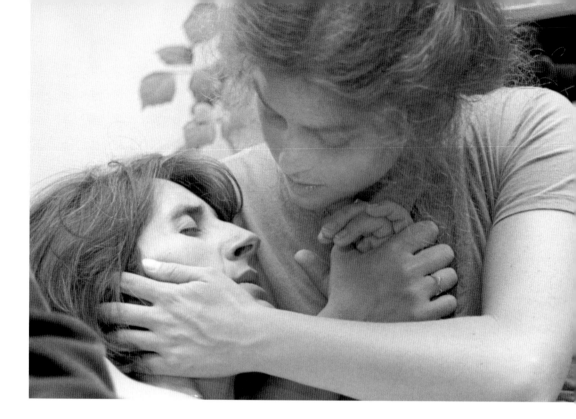

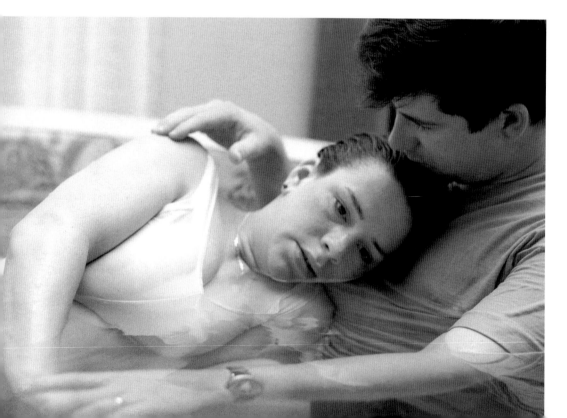

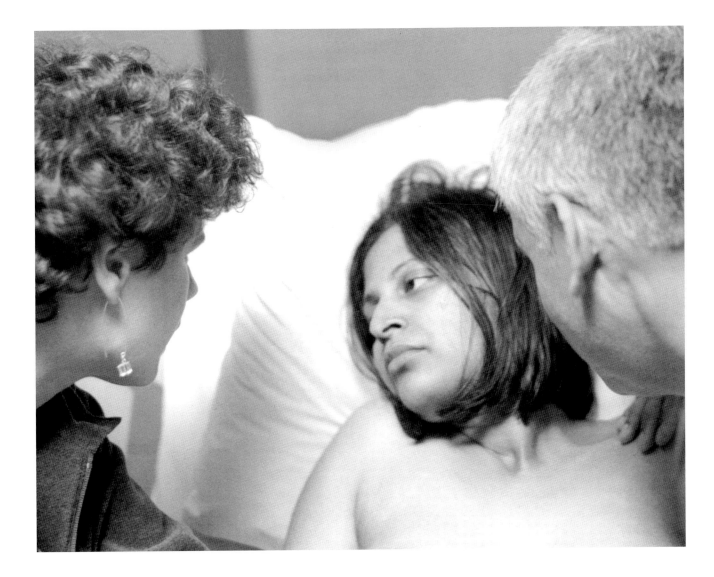

"I FELT EMBRACED WITH THE RELIEF OF PAIN

WHEN THE CONTRACTION WAS OVER."

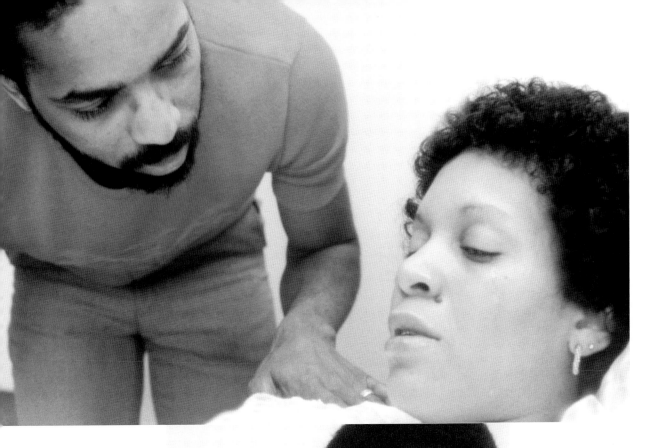

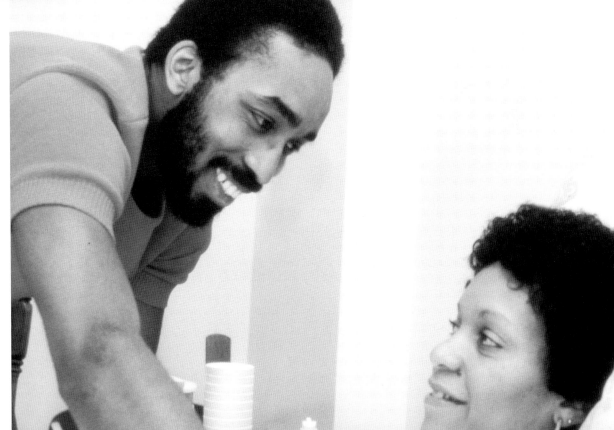

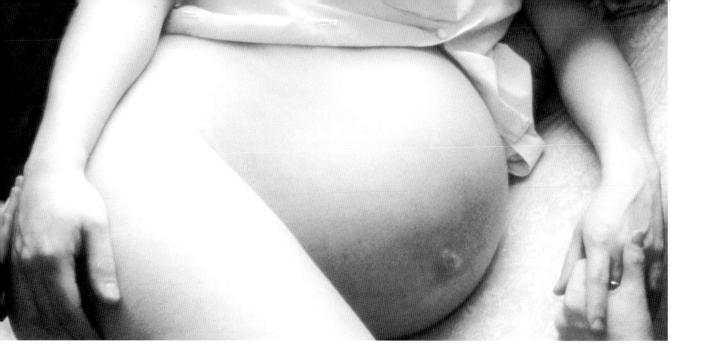

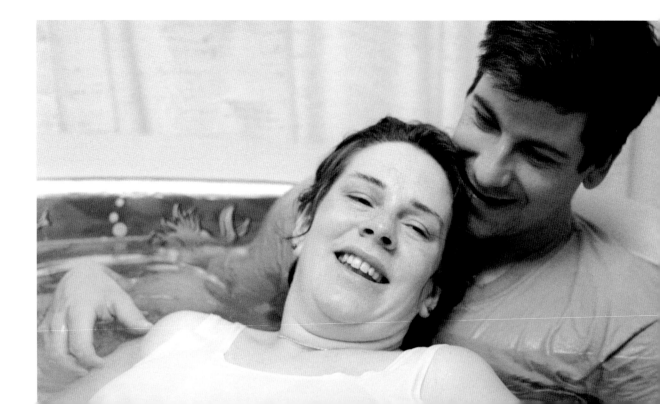

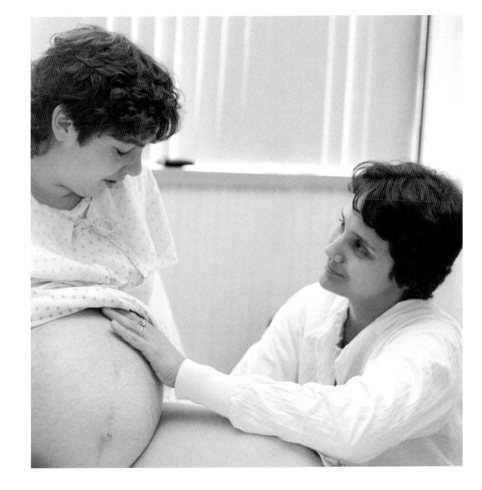

"THE PULL OF GRAVITY. I FELT EARTHBOUND."

"THE CONTRACTIONS, SO PERSISTENT."

"THEY HURT BUT NOTHING'S WRONG."

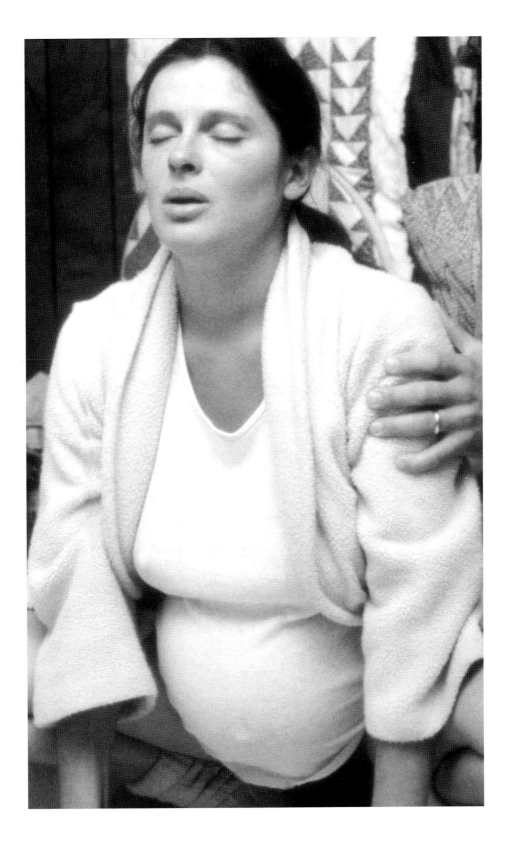

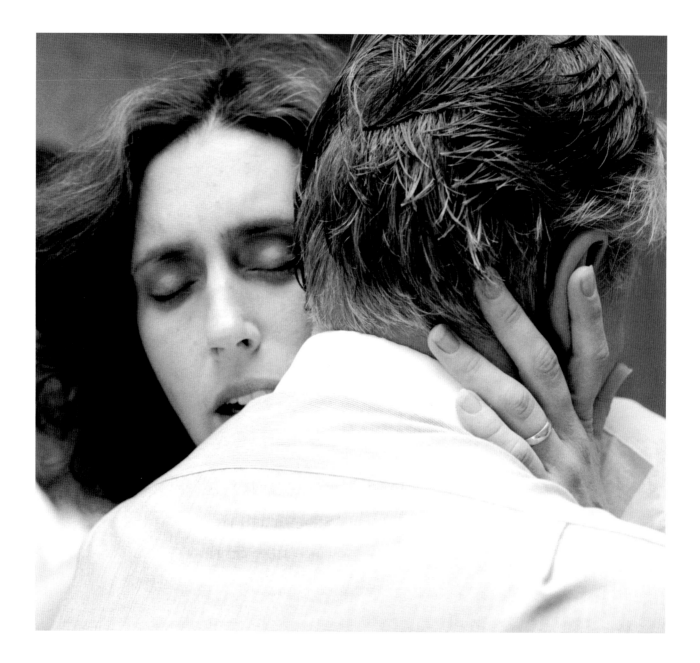

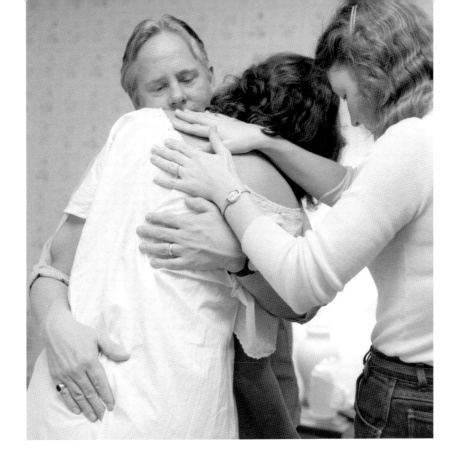

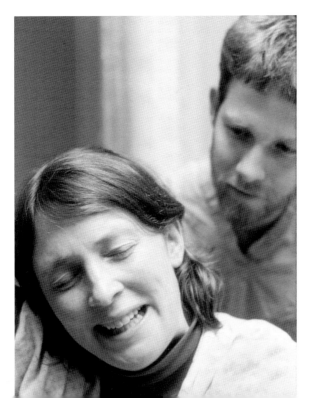

"FEELING I CAN'T DO THIS ANY MORE."

"CHAOS."

"FEELING ANCIENT."

"FINALLY ACCEPTING THAT I HAVE TO DO IT."

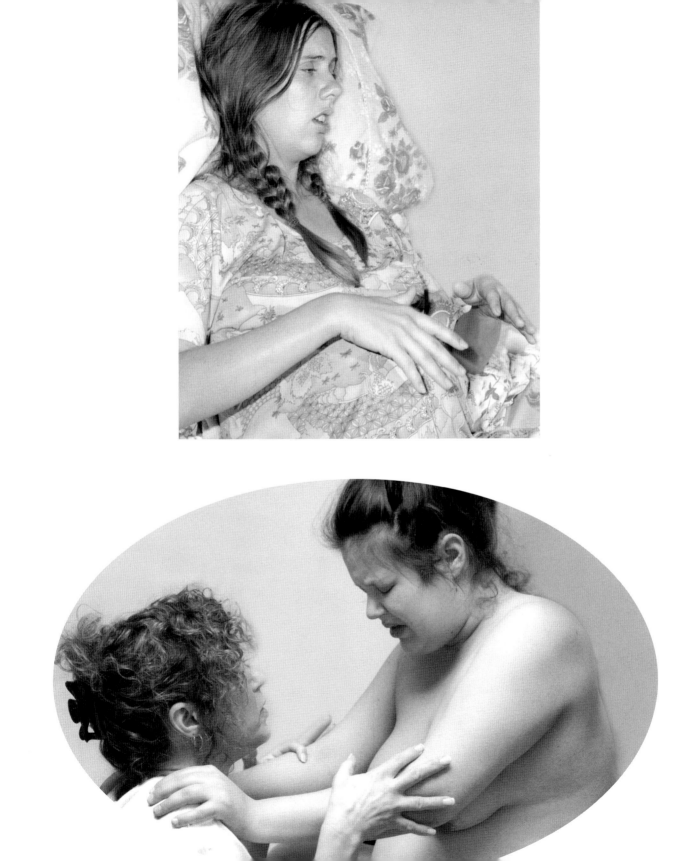

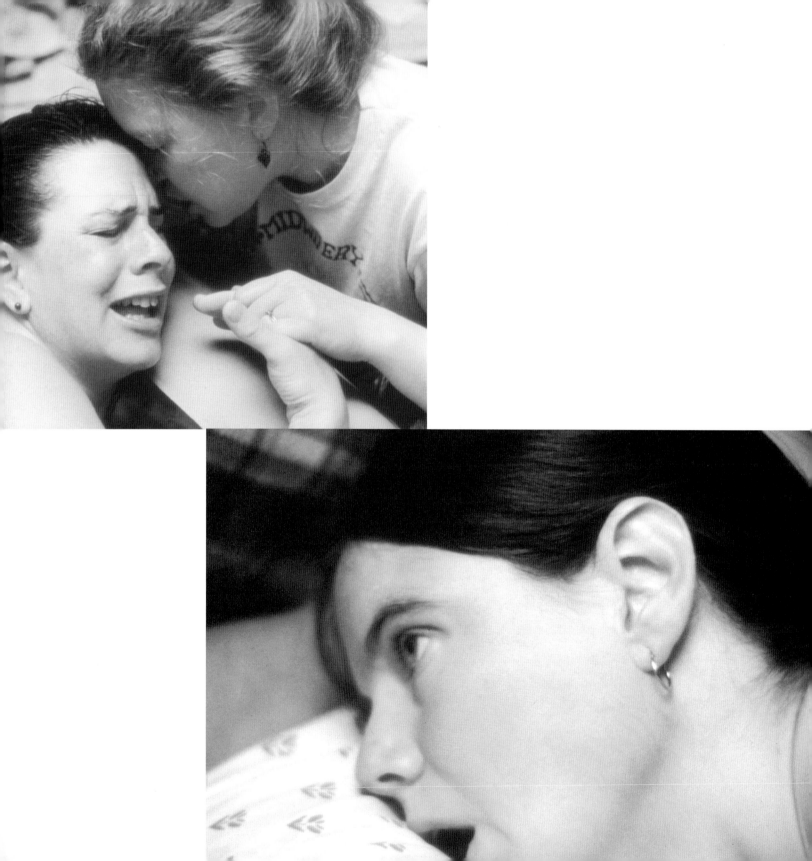

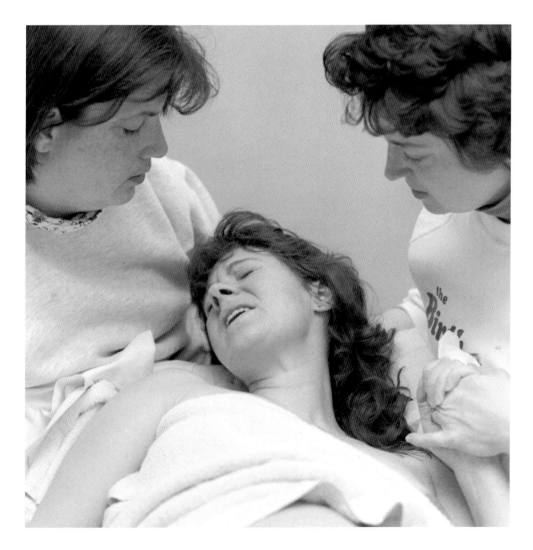

"IT'S A FORCE…YOU CAN'T STOP."

"HAVE TO GO WITH IT."

"I WAS AFRAID BUT I HAD TO OPEN UP."

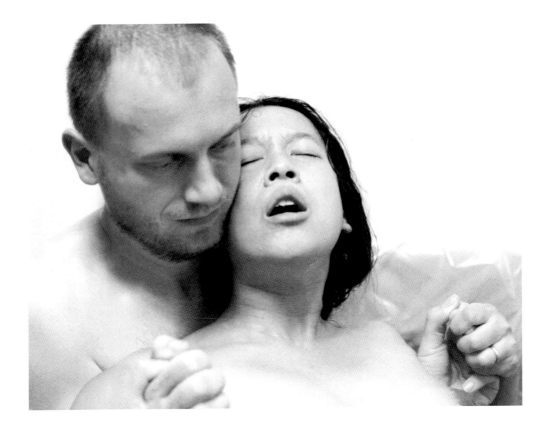

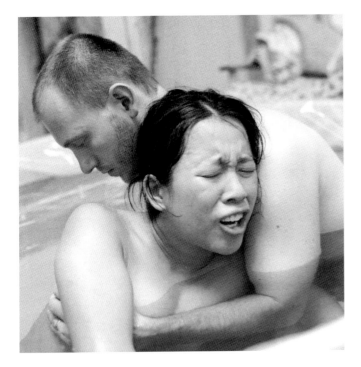

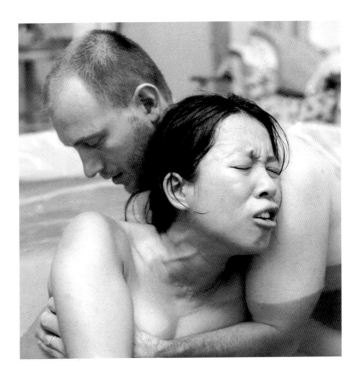

BIRTH

PASSIONATE WITH STRENGTH AND COURAGE,

birthing woman moves another body through her own, past muscle, tissue and bone.

Releasing her embrace of nine months, woman opens in utmost response

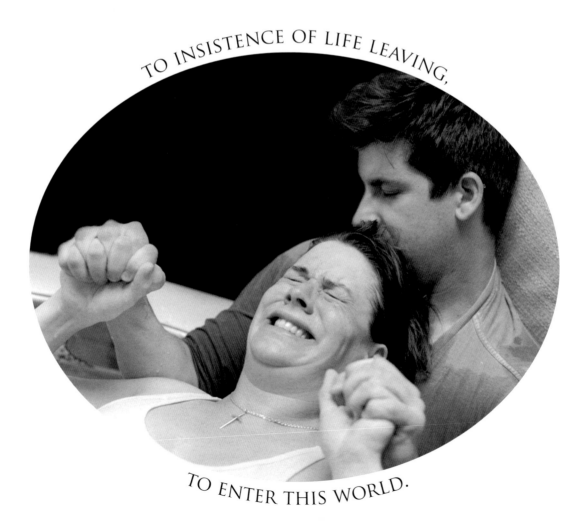

TO INSISTENCE OF LIFE LEAVING,

TO ENTER THIS WORLD.

AND EACH OF US NEWBORNS

crosses a threshold of supreme consequence,

leaving waters of paradise where all needs are met,

to abide in earthly possibilities, uncertainties and responsibilities.

Surrounded by air, we take first breath.

IT LASTS A LIFETIME.

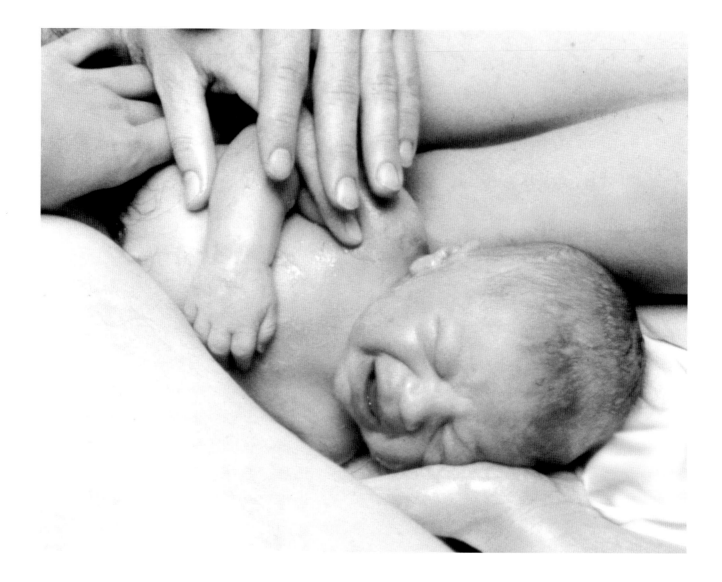

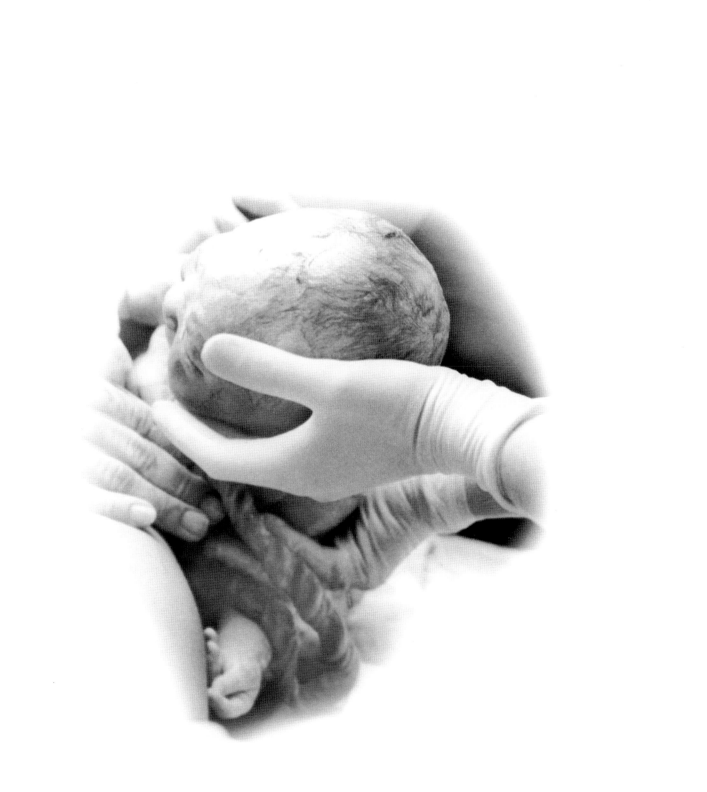

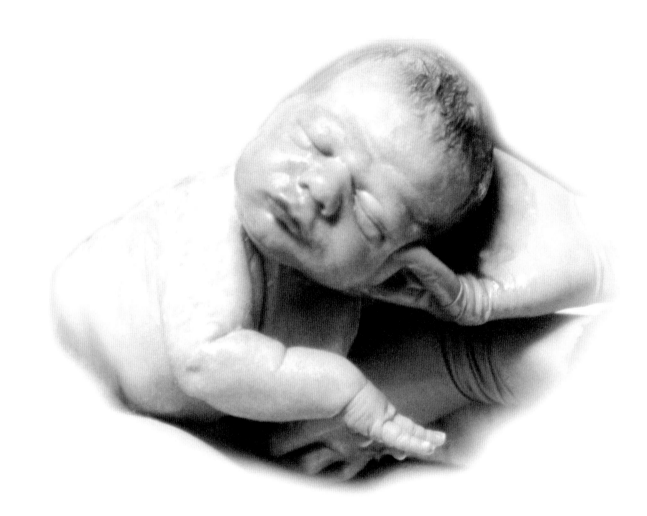

"YOU KNOW BEING BORN IS IMPORTANT TO YOU.
YOU KNOW NOTHING ELSE WAS EVER SO
IMPORTANT TO YOU."

Carl Sandburg

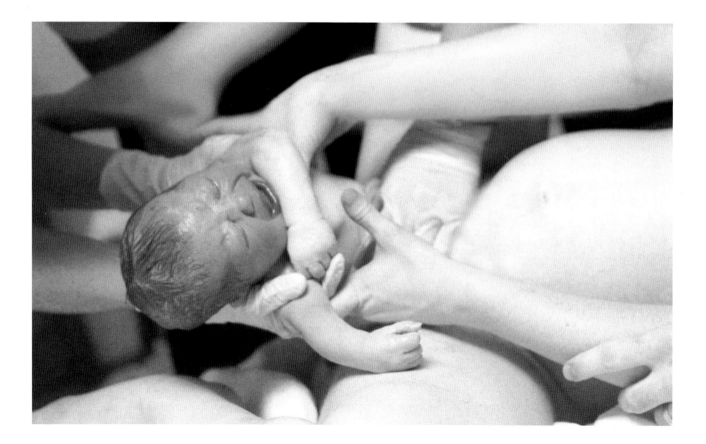

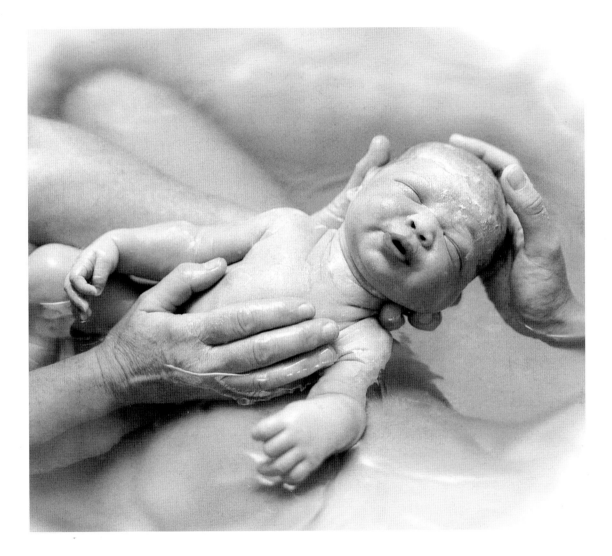

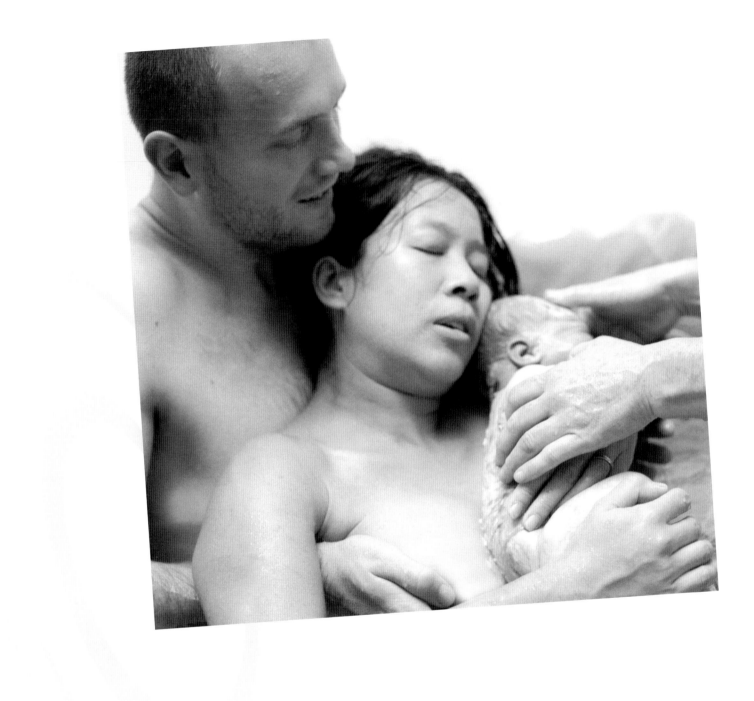

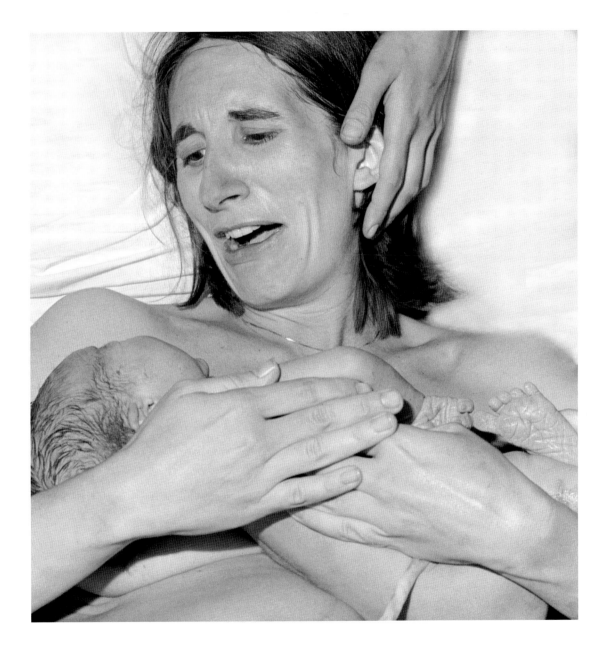

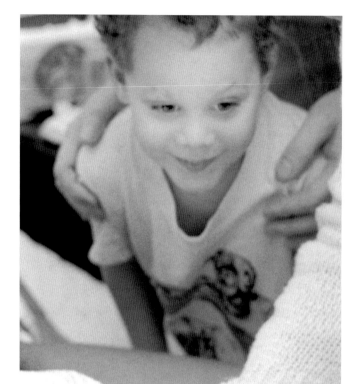

"...THE BABY HOLY WITH POSSIBILITIES,

THAT'S ALL OF US AT BIRTH."

Tillie Olsen

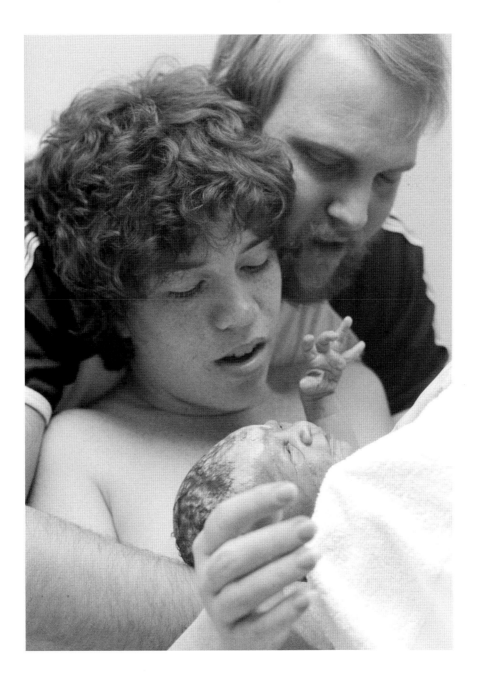

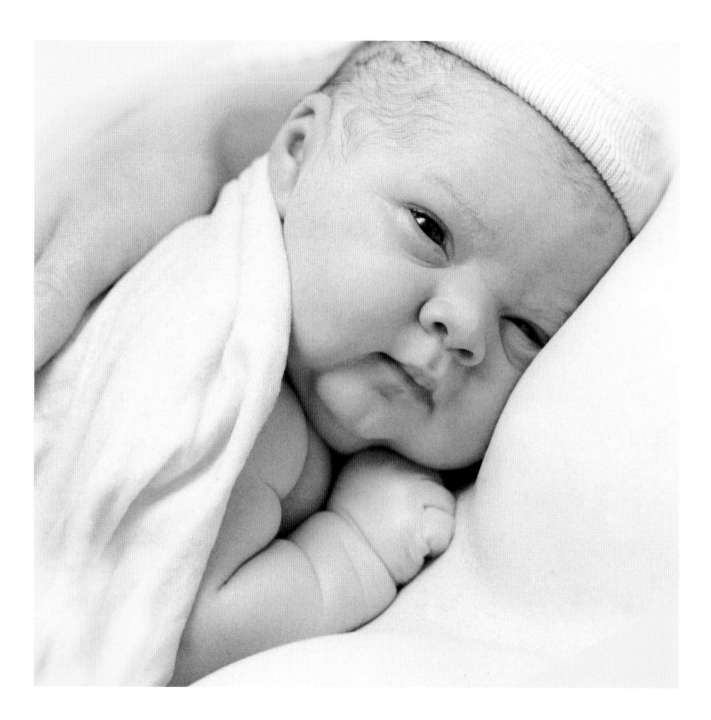

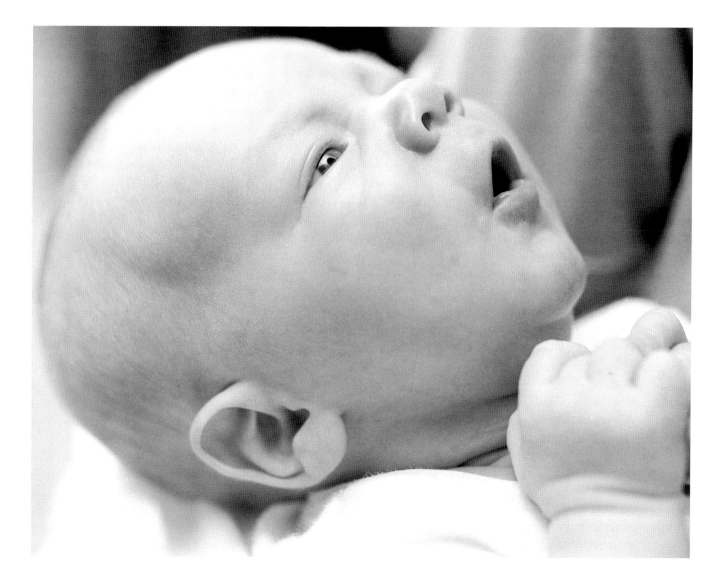

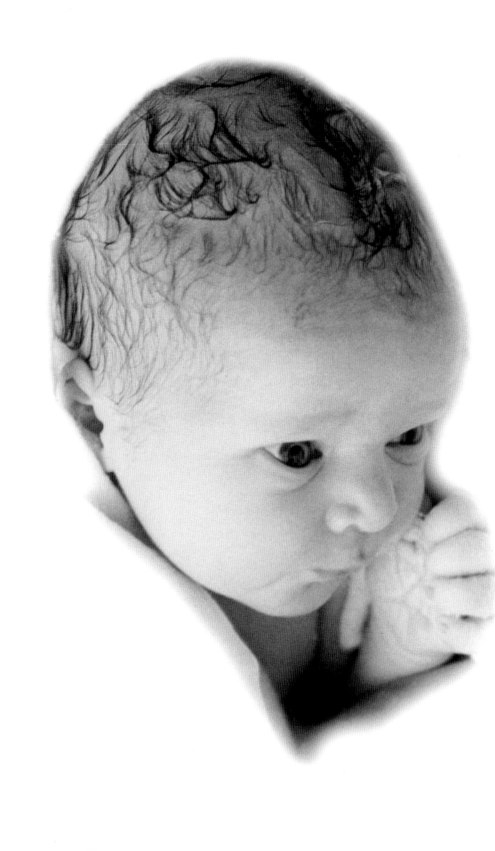

BIRTH

IS AS SAFE
AS LIFE
GETS

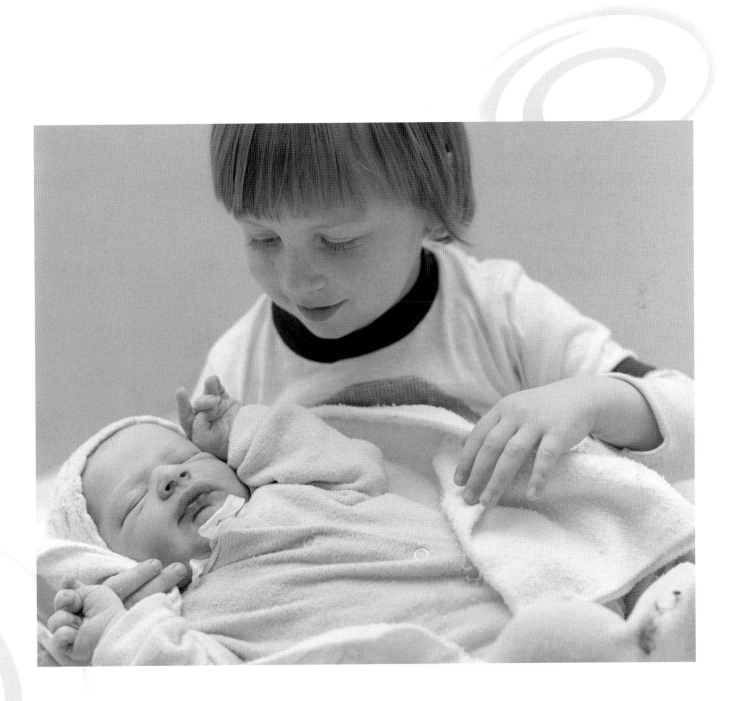

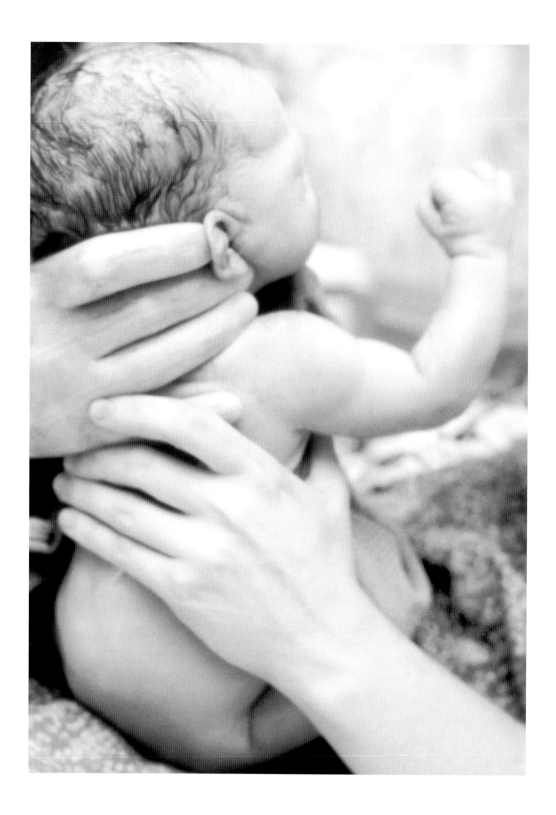

WE THE NEWBORNS

Into Being.

Original and ancient.

Old wisdom in new bodies.

Mystery familiar in our cells and our soul.

Journeying through exquisite terrain,

we come to earth by birth.

With satisfaction and longing,

THE QUESTION IS ASKING.

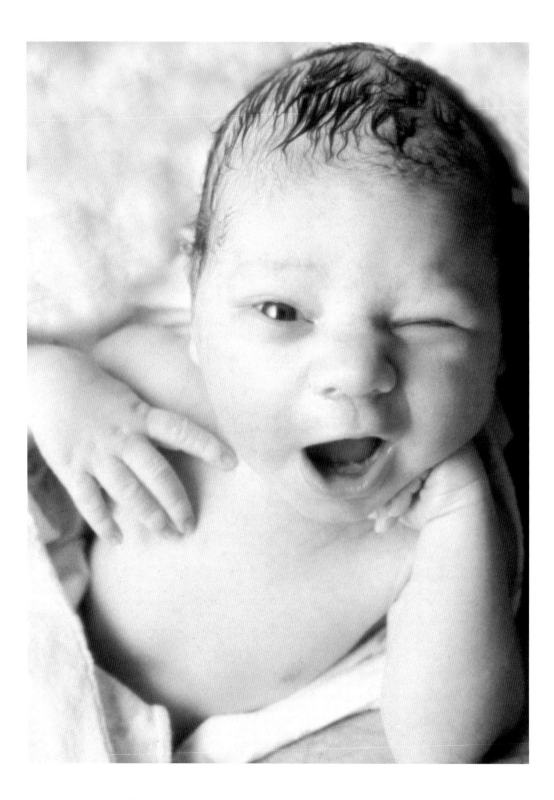

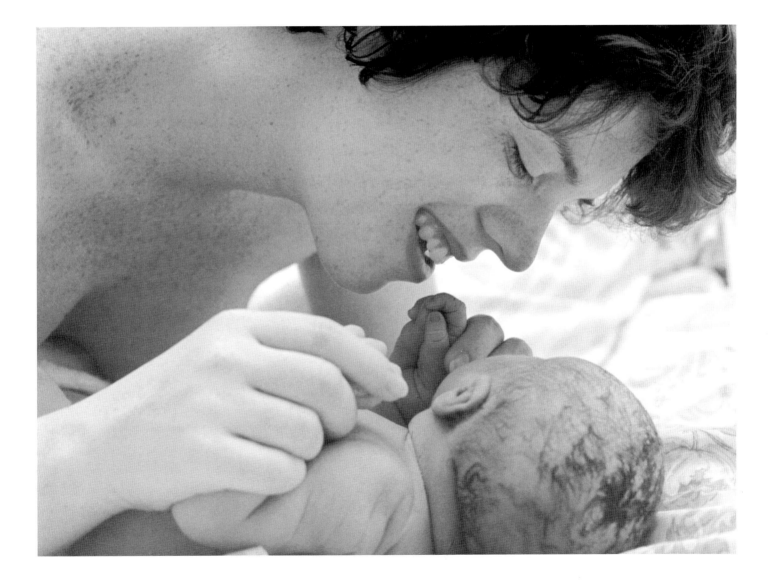

"LOOKING FOR THE FACE I HAD BEFORE THE WORLD WAS BORN."

William Yeats

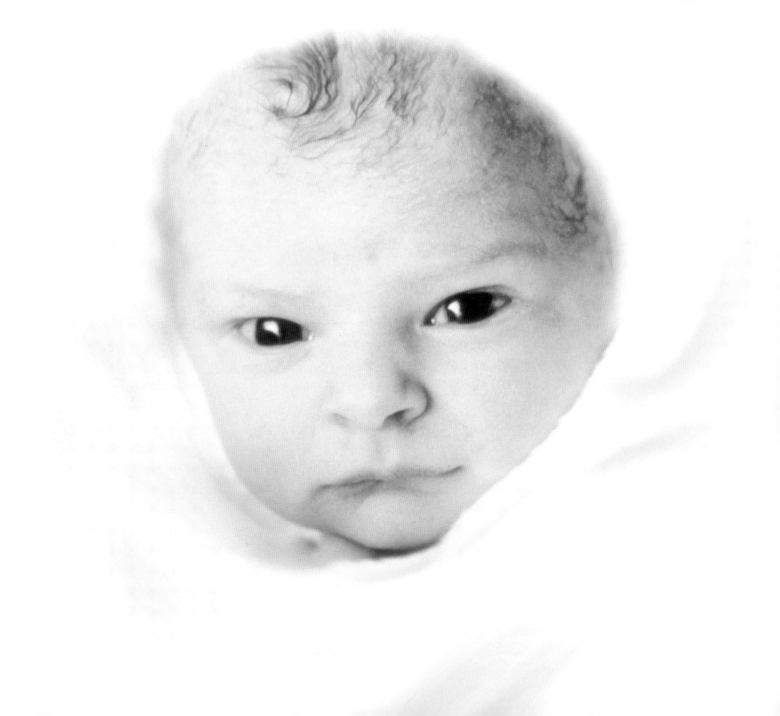

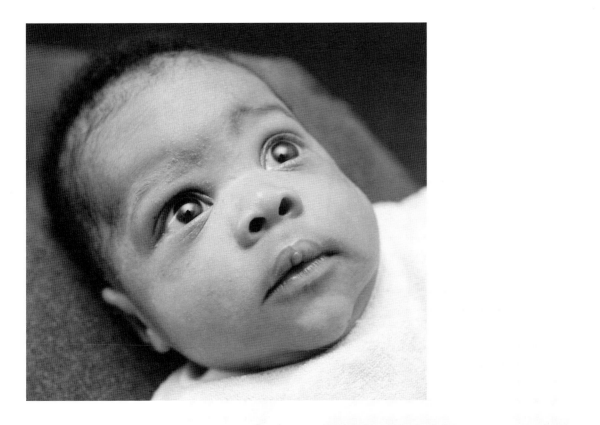

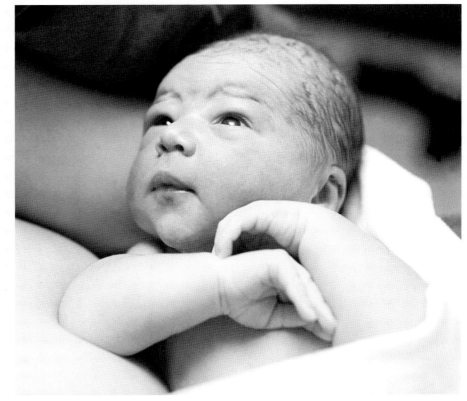

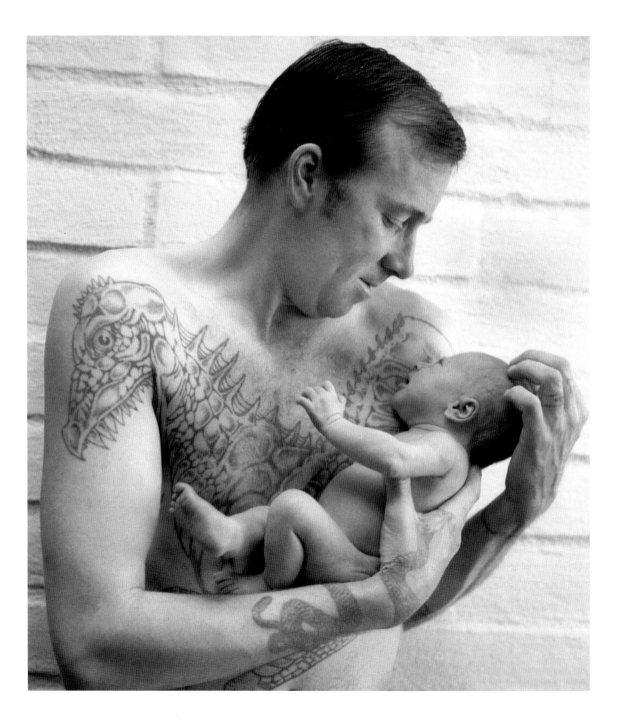

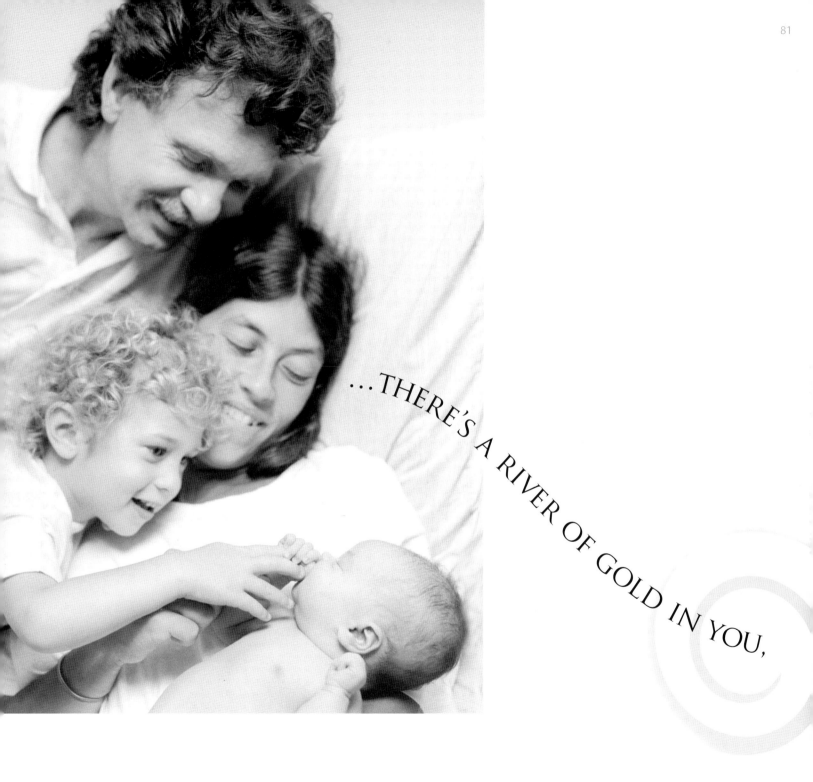

...THERE'S A RIVER OF GOLD IN YOU,

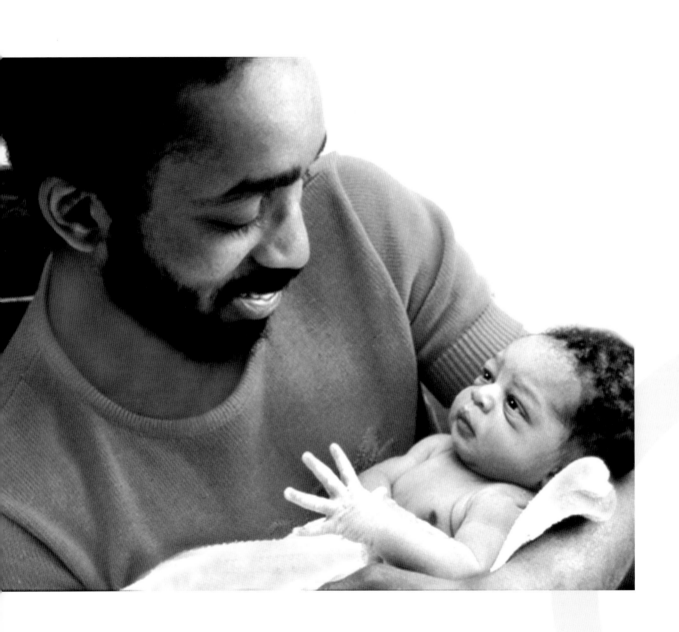

MYSTERIES UNTOLD IN YOU…"

Teri and Robb Singer

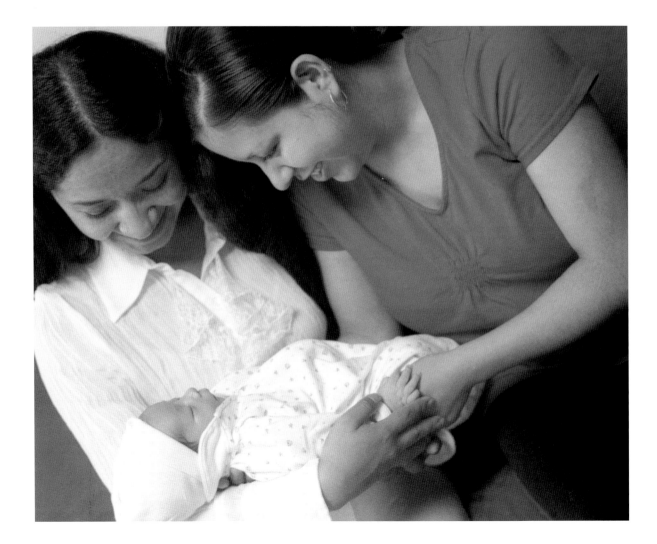

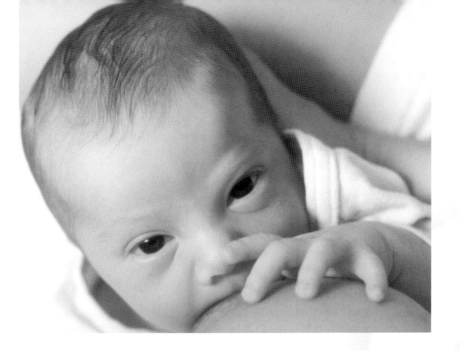

delicious
BEAUTY

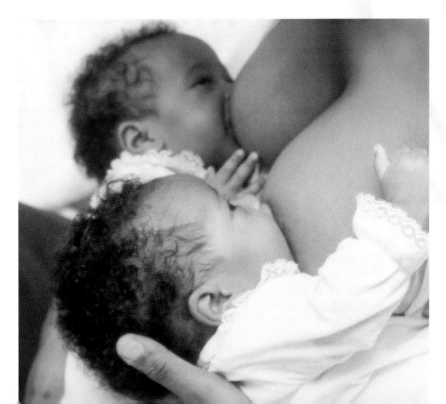

"...WHO ENTERED

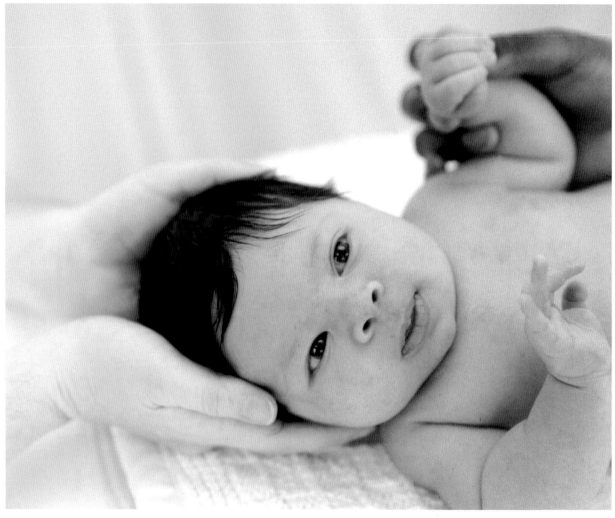

WITHOUT COMING THROUGH THE DOOR,

...WHOSE FEET HAVE NOT

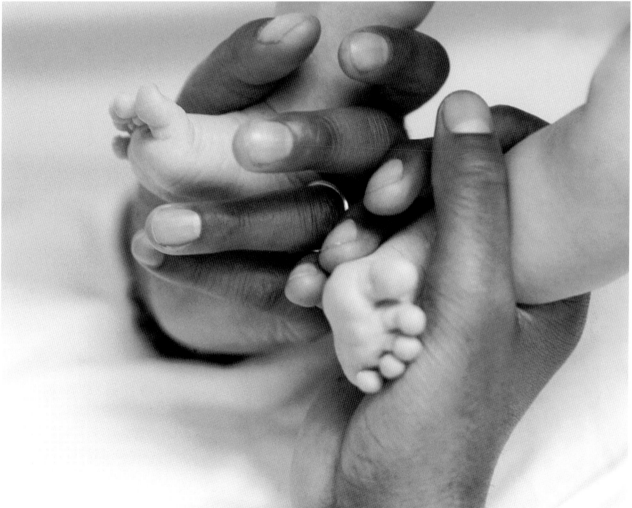

TOUCHED THE GROUND."

Colette

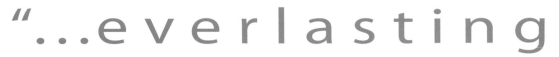

"...everlasting

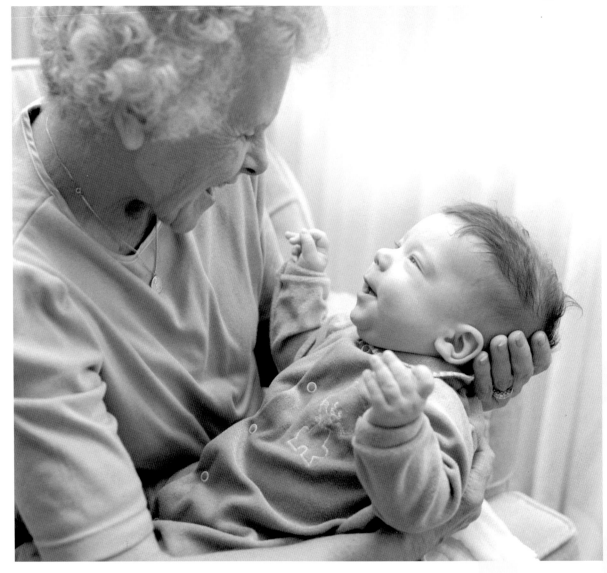

feeling."

Gertrude Stein

WHAT IF...

WE THE NEWBORNS

GAZE INTO OUR OWN EYES
AND INTO THE EYES OF ONE ANOTHER,

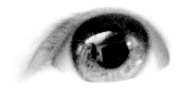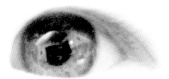

SEEING THE GRACE
OF BIRTH'S POSSIBILITIES?

ABOUT THE AUTHOR

Photographing childbirth since 1975, and expressing the art within this epic experience, has been my path. Along the way I became a midwife. My responsibility to this privileged work is to communicate what I see, hear and learn. I am able to do this by writing, producing photographs and DVDs, teaching and counseling. I feel very grateful for these opportunities.

I invite you to send me your insights, thoughts and experiences about birth to: insight@harriettehartigan.com. Please visit my Web site for more images and ideas exploring this journey of life.

harriettehartigan.com

Here's a birth tote!

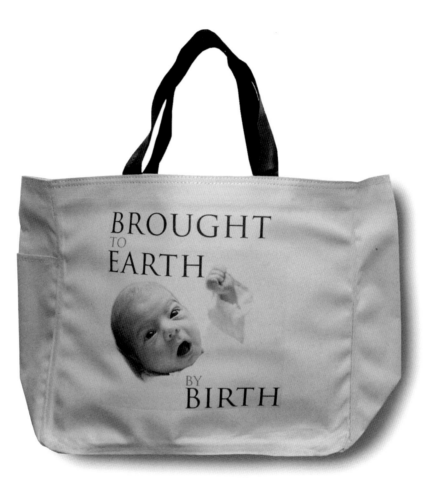

You can find this tote and more stunning birth art and photography by Harriette Hartigan on practical items and in educational resources at:

midwiferytoday.com/products/hhp.htm